A GUIDE TO UNDERSTANDING LISINOPRIL

All You Need to Know About Lisinopril for The Treatment of High Blood Pressure

Dr James Fish

Table of Contents

CHAPTER ONE

What is Lisinopril?

Lisinopril is a drug usually recommended for the treatment of hypertension (hypertension) and cardiovascular breakdown, as well with respect to further developing endurance after a respiratory failure. Angiotensin-converting enzyme (ACE) inhibitors are a class of drugs that work by relaxing blood vessels, allowing blood to flow more easily.

Lisinopril works by inhibiting the angiotensin-converting enzyme, which is a component of the renin-angiotensin-aldosterone system (RAAS) in the body. The fluid balance and blood pressure are controlled by this system. Lisinopril prevents the formation of angiotensin II, which is a substance that narrows blood vessels and releases hormones like aldosterone that can raise blood pressure. It does this by blocking this enzyme. Accordingly, lisinopril assists with bringing down pulse, decline the responsibility on the heart, and work on the heart's productivity in siphoning blood.

The medication is typically taken once daily, either with or without food, as a tablet. The condition being treated and the patient's response to the medication influence the dosage. Normal results of lisinopril incorporate hack, unsteadiness, cerebral pain, weariness, and sickness. Kidney issues, elevated potassium levels, and severe allergic reactions are among the more serious side effects, though they are less common.

Lisinopril can have an effect on kidney function and electrolyte levels, so patients must be closely monitored. Patients must adhere to their physician's instructions and report any unusual symptoms or side effects. When taken as directed, lisinopril is frequently used in clinical practice and is generally regarded as safe and effective. Be that as it may, it isn't prescribed for use during pregnancy because of expected damage to the creating hatchling.

CHAPTER TWO

Method of operation

Lisinopril, an angiotensin-changing over protein (Pro) inhibitor, fundamentally works by repressing the movement of the compound Pro. This chemical assumes a vital part in the renin-angiotensin-aldosterone framework (RAAS), which controls circulatory strain and liquid equilibrium in the body.

Angiotensin I, an inactive precursor, is transformed by ACE into angiotensin II, a potent vasoconstrictor, under normal physiological conditions. There are several significant effects of angiotensin II: It stimulates the adrenal glands to release aldosterone and makes blood vessels narrow, which raises blood pressure. Aldosterone advances sodium and water maintenance by the kidneys, further expanding blood volume and, thusly, circulatory strain.

The inhibition of ACE, which reduces the conversion of angiotensin I to angiotensin II, is the mechanism of action of lisinopril. Several therapeutic effects result from this:

Vasodilation: Lisinopril lowers blood pressure by reducing angiotensin II levels, which causes blood vessels to dilate (widen). By lowering the resistance against which the heart must pump, this vasodilatory effect reduces the heart's workload.

Reduced Production of Aldosterone: Aldosterone secretion is reduced when angiotensin II levels are lower. This prompts less sodium and water maintenance by the kidneys, which diminishes blood volume and further brings down circulatory strain.

Reduced Activity of the Sympathetic Nervous System:

Angiotensin II can invigorate the thoughtful sensory system, which increments pulse and circulatory strain. By restraining its arrangement, lisinopril lessens these impacts.

Lisinopril's effectiveness as a treatment for heart failure and hypertension is bolstered by the combination of these effects. Lisinopril can also help patients who have had a heart attack survive by reducing the workload on the heart and increasing blood flow. The general outcome is better administration of circulatory strain, further developed heart capability, and improved cardiovascular wellbeing.

CHAPTER THREE

Conditions treated by lisinopril

Lisinopril is a flexible medicine that essentially treats three key circumstances: management of hypertension, heart failure, and post-myocardial infarction (also known as a heart attack). Its adequacy around there originates from its job as an angiotensin-changing over compound (ACE) inhibitor, which directs pulse and backing cardiovascular wellbeing.

Hypertension

Hypertension, or hypertension, is one of the most widely recognized conditions treated with lisinopril. Lisinopril helps lower blood pressure by inhibiting the conversion of angiotensin I to angiotensin II. This helps relax the blood vessels. Because it helps prevent complications like stroke, heart attack, and kidney problems, lowering high blood pressure is essential. To achieve optimal blood pressure control, lisinopril is frequently prescribed either on its own or in conjunction with other antihypertensive medications.

Heart Failure Lisinopril is also used to treat heart failure, a condition in which the heart is unable to effectively pump blood to meet the body's requirements. Lisinopril reduces the strain on the heart by reducing the production of angiotensin II. This improves cardiac output and reduces symptoms of heart failure like shortness of breath, fatigue, and leg and ankle swelling. Lisinopril also helps prevent fluid retention, a common issue in heart failure patients, by lowering aldosterone levels.

Management of Post-Myocardial Infarction A heart attack can significantly weaken the heart muscle. During the recovery phase, lisinopril is frequently prescribed to help increase survival rates and prevent further damage. By bringing down circulatory strain and decreasing the responsibility on the heart, lisinopril upholds the mending system and forestalls future cardiovascular occasions. By stabilizing cardiovascular function and lowering the likelihood of subsequent heart attacks, its use in post-myocardial infarction patients has the potential to improve long-term outcomes.

CHAPTER FOUR

Advantages of Lisinopril

Because of its numerous advantages, lisinopril is frequently prescribed for cardiovascular and renal conditions. Its function as an angiotensin-converting enzyme (ACE) inhibitor, which helps control blood pressure and improve heart and kidney health, is where its primary advantages lie.

Controlling High Blood Pressure Lisinopril is very good at lowering hypertension, which is a major risk factor for cardiovascular diseases. Lisinopril causes vasodilation, or the widening of blood vessels, by inhibiting the formation of angiotensin II, a substance that makes blood vessels narrow. This lowers blood pressure, lowering the likelihood of complications like kidney damage, heart attack, and stroke.

Lisinopril reduces blood pressure and promotes improved cardiac output in patients with heart failure, thereby easing the burden on the heart. Patients' quality of life is improved as a result of this, which helps alleviate symptoms like fatigue, shortness of breath, and swelling. Additionally, it may increase survival rates and reduce hospitalizations for heart failure exacerbations.

Patients recovering from a myocardial infarction (heart attack) can benefit from taking lisinopril. By easing the burden on the heart and preventing further damage, it contributes to an increase in survival rates. This reduces the likelihood of future heart attacks and improves long-term outcomes.

Protection of the Kidneys Lisinopril protects the kidneys, particularly in diabetics and those with chronic kidney disease. It aids in sloweding the progression of kidney damage by lowering blood pressure and reducing proteinuria, or excessive protein in the urine. Patients with diabetes who are at a high risk of developing diabetic nephropathy need to pay close attention to this.

The majority of patients tolerate lisinopril well and find it convenient. Coughing and dizziness are two common side effects that are typically mild and manageable. As a once-daily oral tablet, it is also easy to use, which helps patients stick to their medication plan.

Versatility Lisinopril is a useful medication in clinical practice because it can be used off-label to treat diabetic nephropathy as well as treat hypertension, heart failure, and post-heart attack management. Patients who have cardiovascular and renal conditions at the same time benefit from this multifaceted utility by streamlining their treatment plans.

Lisinopril is a key component in the treatment of hypertension, heart failure, and post-myocardial infarction care due to its overall advantages in enhancing patient outcomes, protecting renal function, and improving cardiovascular health.

CHAPTER FIVE

Dosing

Lisinopril comes in a variety of tablet strengths, typically ranging from 2.5 mg to 40 mg, for oral administration. Lisinopril dosages are determined by the patient's response to the medication, the condition being treated, and their overall health. A comprehensive overview of its administration and dosing is as follows:

Hypertension The initial dose of lisinopril for the treatment of hypertension is typically 10 mg once daily. The usual maintenance dose, which ranges from 20 mg to 40 mg once daily, can be adjusted based on the response of the patient to the medication. A lower starting dose of 2.5 mg to 5 mg may be used for patients who are sensitive to ACE inhibitors or have a high risk of renal impairment.

Heart Failure To prevent a rapid drop in blood pressure, the initial dose of heart failure medication is frequently decreased. The usual starting dose is 2.5 mg to 5 mg once daily. Depending on the patient's tolerance and clinical response, the dose may be gradually increased. Typically, the recommended daily maintenance dose is between 20 and 40 mg.

Lisinopril is administered at a low dose following a heart attack to determine tolerance. In most cases, the first dose is 5 mg within 24 hours of the occurrence, followed by another 5 mg dose within 24 hours, and finally 10 mg once per day. Depending on the patient's condition and response, the dose can be changed up to 20 mg once daily.

Unique Populaces

Renal Disability: Lisinopril doses are adjusted based on creatinine clearance levels in renally impaired patients. For moderate to serious renal weakness, the underlying portion might be all around as low as 2.5 mg to keep away from over the top gathering of the medication.

Elderly: Older patients might require lower beginning portions because of the potential for diminished renal capability and a higher aversion to the medication.

CHAPTER SIX
Contraindications

Lisinopril, similar to all meds, has explicit contraindications that should be considered prior to endorsing it. Lisinopril should not be used in certain patients due to the presence of these contraindications, which are conditions or factors that raise the risk of adverse effects.

Due to the possibility of fetal toxicity, pregnant women should not take lisinopril, especially in the second and third trimesters. Lisinopril and other ACE inhibitors can harm or even kill the developing fetus. Lisinopril should be stopped as soon as possible and an alternative medication should be used if pregnancy is detected during treatment.

Angioedema This medication should not be used by patients who have had angioedema as a result of previous treatment with an ACE inhibitor, such as lisinopril. A severe allergic reaction known as angioedema is characterized by swelling of the face, lips, tongue, and occasionally the throat. This swelling can obstruct the airways and be life-threatening.

Hyperkalemia Patients with hyperkalemia (high potassium levels) should not take lisinopril. This medication may raise potassium levels, which could cause dangerous arrhythmias in the heart. Patients with conditions that incline them toward hyperkalemia, for example, certain kidney issues or those taking potassium-saving diuretics or potassium supplements, ought to keep away from lisinopril.

Patients with Severe Renal Impairment Although lisinopril is frequently used to maintain kidney function in patients with mild to moderate renal impairment, it is contraindicated in patients with severe renal impairment and dialysis patients. Due to decreased renal clearance, these patients are at a greater risk of accumulating the drug and developing potential toxicity.

Lisinopril should not be taken by people who have bilateral renal artery stenosis, which is a narrowing of the arteries that supply both kidneys. The medication may further impair renal blood flow and function in such instances, which could result in acute renal failure.

Hypersensitivity Patients who are known to be allergic to lisinopril or any of its components should not take this medication. Anaphylaxis to severe rashes are all examples of allergic reactions.

Lisinopril is approved for the treatment of hypertension in children, but it should be used with caution and under close medical supervision. It has not been proven to be safe or effective for children under the age of six.

Aortic Stenosis: Other Factors to Consider Lisinopril can cause hypotension, so patients with aortic stenosis or other forms of outflow obstruction should exercise caution.

Liver Infection: Lisinopril metabolism may be altered in patients with severe liver disease, necessitating close observation and possible dose adjustments.

Lisinopril is a profoundly viable medicine for some patients, yet it is fundamental to consider these contraindications to stay away from serious unfriendly impacts. Legitimate patient assessment and observing are essential to guaranteeing protected and successful utilization of lisinopril.

CHAPTER SEVEN

Combinations with Other Drugs

An ACE inhibitor like lisinopril can interact with other medications, which could change how well it works or make it more likely to cause side effects. Important interactions to keep an eye on include:

Diuretics

Thiazide and Circle Diuretics: Simultaneous use with lisinopril can prompt unreasonable pulse decrease, causing hypotension. Lisinopril should be taken at lower doses at first in patients who are already taking diuretics to avoid this risk.

Supplements and diuretics low in potassium: When combined with lisinopril, these can raise the risk of hyperkalemia. It's important to keep an eye on potassium levels.

Nonsteroidal Mitigating Medications (NSAIDs)

NSAIDs, including ibuprofen and naproxen, can lessen the antihypertensive impact of lisinopril and increment the gamble of kidney harm. This is especially important for people who already have kidney problems or are dehydrated.

Lithium

Lisinopril can increment serum lithium levels, possibly prompting lithium poisonousness. Tremors, confusion, and renal dysfunction are all signs of lithium toxicity. When these drugs are taken together, lithium levels need to be checked on a regular basis.

Beta-blockers, calcium channel blockers, and other vascular dilators are additional antihypertensive medications. Together with lisinopril, these can have additive effects that can raise the risk of hypotension. Dose adjustments and careful monitoring may be required.

Insulin and oral hypoglycemics: Antidiabetic medications Lisinopril may increase these medications' ability to lower blood glucose, which could lead to hypoglycemia. When starting or adjusting their doses of lisinopril, patients should closely monitor their blood glucose levels.

Gold Injections Lisinopril can occasionally interact with gold injections, which are used in some cases of rheumatoid arthritis. Nausea, vomiting, and hypotension are all signs of this reaction, which is called a nitritoid reaction.

Immunosuppressants and Cytotoxic Specialists

Azathioprine and Cyclophosphamide: Simultaneous use with lisinopril might expand the gamble of hematologic aftereffects like leukopenia (decrease in white platelets). Monitoring of blood counts on a regular basis is advised.

Lisinopril's blood pressure-lowering effects can be exacerbated and the risk of fainting or dizziness can rise when taking alcohol with the medication.

Lisinopril and angiotensin receptor blockers (ARBs) or direct renin inhibitors (like aliskiren) can increase the risk of hyperkalemia, hypotension, and renal impairment when taken together. This mix is for the most part kept away from except if totally essential and under severe clinical oversight.

CHAPTER EIGHT

Potential Side Effects

Lisinopril can have side effects just like any other medication. Despite the fact that most patients tolerate it well, some may experience side effects. These aftereffects can go from gentle to extreme and fluctuate in recurrence.

Common Symptoms of Cough: One of the most common adverse effects of lisinopril is a persistent dry cough, affecting up to 10% of patients. This is because bradykinin, a substance that ACE inhibitors prevent from breaking down, has built up.

Lightheadedness and dizziness: Lisinopril's ability to lower blood pressure is the cause of these symptoms, which are especially noticeable when the medication is first started or when the dose is increased.

Headache: As the body adjusts to the medication, headaches may lessen in frequency.

Fatigue: A general sense of weakness or exhaustion may occur in some patients.

More uncommon Incidental effects

Hyperkalemia: Raised potassium levels can happen, particularly in patients with renal weakness or those taking potassium supplements. Side effects incorporate muscle shortcoming, weariness, and sporadic pulses.

Hypotension: Patients who are dehydrated or taking diuretics are particularly susceptible to experiencing symptoms such as dizziness, fainting, and blurred vision from excessively low blood pressure.

Damage to the kidneys: Even though lisinopril is taken to

protect kidney function, it can sometimes cause or exacerbate renal impairment, especially in people who already have kidney problems.

Elevated serum creatinine and blood urea nitrogen (BUN): These frequently require monitoring and may indicate impaired kidney function.

Angioedema, a rare but serious side effect: Swelling of the face, lips, tongue, and throat is the result of this severe allergic reaction, which may cause breathing difficulties and necessitate immediate medical attention.

Liver Insufficiency: Lisinopril can occasionally cause problems with the liver, such as elevated liver enzymes and, in extreme cases, liver failure. Abdominal pain, dark urine, and jaundice are some of the symptoms.

Neutropenia/Agranulocytosis: White blood cell counts are dangerously low in these conditions, which raises the likelihood of infection. Patients with certain autoimmune diseases and those taking immunosuppressive medication are particularly at risk from this.

Reactions from Allergies: Itching, a rash, and in severe cases, anaphylaxis, a life-threatening allergic reaction that requires immediate treatment, are some of the symptoms.

Effects on the digestive system: Nausea, vomiting, and diarrhea Although they are less common, these side effects can occur and frequently subside as the body adjusts to the medication.

Taste disturbances and other side effects: A metallic or salty taste may be experienced by some patients.

Sensitivity to sunlight has increased: Exaggerated reactions to sunburns can result from photosensitivity.

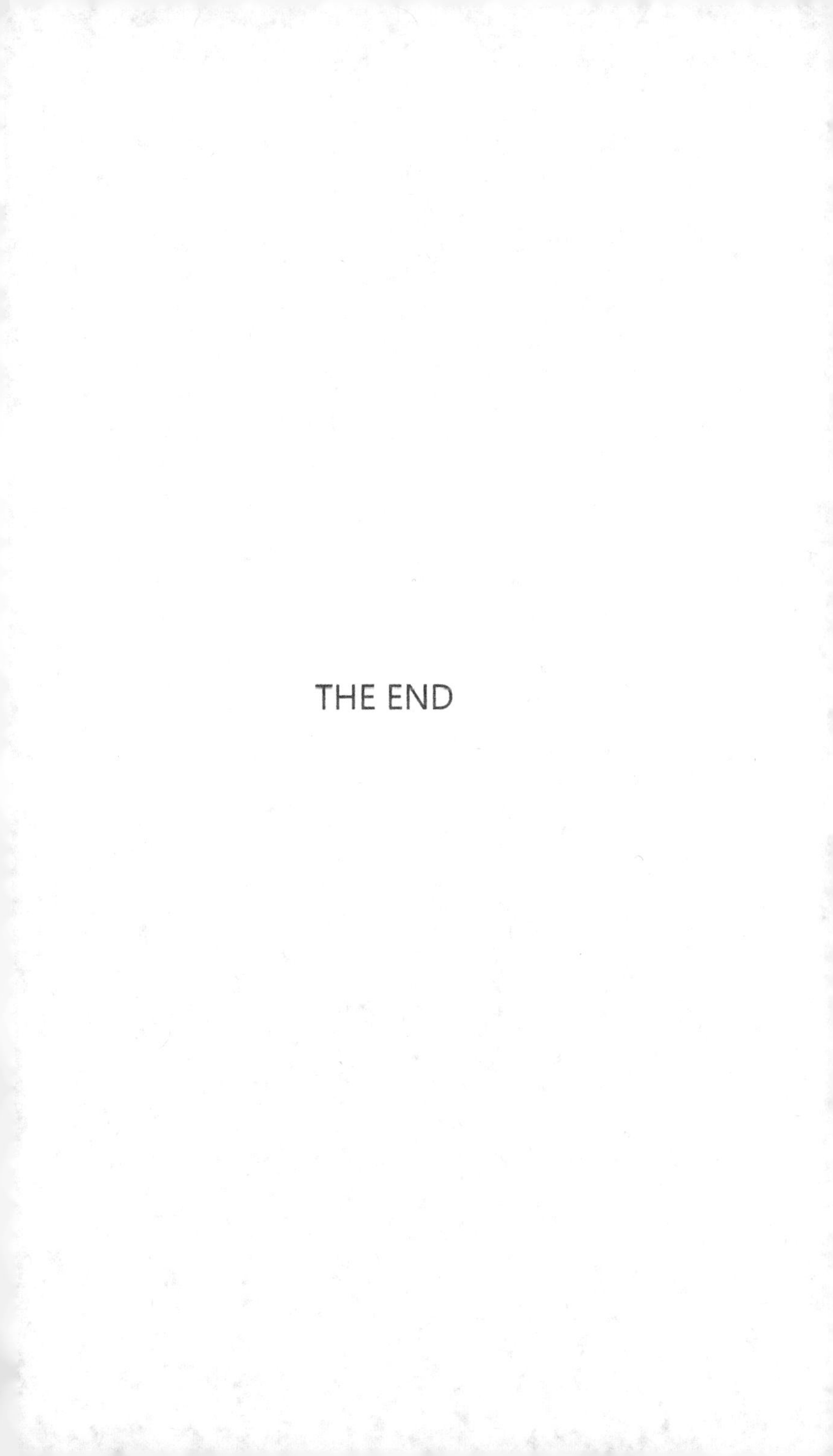

THE END